GLORIOUSTINA ESSIA

HERBAL HARMONY
EMPOWERING WOMEN'S HEALTH NATURALLY

This book was professionally typeset on Reedsy.
Find out more at reedsy.com

Contents

INTRODUCTION

"Herbal Harmony: Empowering Women's Health Naturally" is a heartfelt invitation to every woman who seeks a deeper connection with her body and the natural world. This book is about rediscovering the ancient wisdom of herbal medicine and how it can support the unique health journey of women at all stages of life.

Women's wellness is beautifully complex, marked by cycles that ebb and flow like the tides. It's a journey that intertwines physical, emotional, and spiritual health, requiring care that understands and honors these intricacies. For generations, herbal medicine has been a trusted ally for women, offering gentle yet powerful support that aligns with the body's natural rhythms and healing capabilities.

In this guide, we'll explore the rich tradition of using herbs for health and healing, stretching back through history and across cultures. The tradition recognizes the body's wisdom and seeks to support it with nature's bounty. From easing menstrual cramps to helping pregnancy, from navigating the shifts of menopause to enhancing beauty and well-being, herbs have been there, providing balance, relief, and nourishment.

But this book is more than just a collection of herbal remedies. It's an invitation to engage with nature's healing power in an informed, intuitive, and deeply personal way. We'll learn how to listen to our bodies and respond with care that is as nurturing as it is effective. We'll discover how integrating herbs into our daily lives can profoundly change our health and happiness.

Herbal medicine offers a path to wellness that is both empowering and enriching, allowing us to take our health into our own hands naturally. It's an approach that treats symptoms and nurtures overall well-being, honoring the body's ability to heal and thrive.

As we journey through these pages, we'll uncover the secrets of nature's pharmacy, learning how to use herbs to address specific health concerns and enhance our overall quality of life. This is a journey of transformation, coming back to our roots, and finding harmony within ourselves and the natural world.

So, whether you're new to herbal medicine or looking to deepen your practice, "Herbal Harmony" guides you. Together, we'll explore how herbs can support, heal, and celebrate the incredible journey of being a woman. Welcome to a world where your health and well-being are in harmony with nature.

CHAPTER 1: THE FOUNDATION OF HERBAL MEDICINE FOR WOMEN

The journey into herbal medicine for women is as ancient as it is profound, deeply rooted in the understanding that nature holds the key to nurturing health, balance, and vitality. This chapter lays the groundwork for a transformative exploration of how herbs can be harnessed to support women's health across all stages of life. It is a testament to the power of the natural world and its capacity to heal, soothe, and empower.

Understanding Herbal Medicine

Herbal medicine is the art and science of using plants for therapeutic purposes. It encompasses a holistic approach, considering health's physical, emotional, and spiritual aspects. This approach offers women a way to align with the body's natural rhythms and address specific health concerns with gentleness and respect. With their complex biochemical makeup, herbs can provide targeted support for hormonal balance, reproductive health, and emotional well-being.

The efficacy of herbal medicine is rooted in centuries of traditional use, supported increasingly by contemporary scientific research. This rich tapestry of knowledge provides a solid foundation for understanding how different herbs work and how they can be used safely and effectively.

Safety Guidelines for Using Herbs

While herbs are natural, their potent medicinal properties mean they must be used with care and respect. Understanding dosages, potential side effects, and contraindications is crucial, especially for pregnant or breastfeeding women, those with existing health conditions, or anyone taking prescription medications.

- **Consultation with Healthcare Providers:** Always discuss herbal remedies with a healthcare provider, particularly if you have pre-existing conditions or are taking other medications.
- **Quality and Purity of Herbs:** Source herbs from reputable suppliers to ensure they are free from contaminants and accurately labeled.
- **Start with Low Doses:** Begin with the lowest possible dose to see how your body responds, gradually increasing as needed under professional guidance.

Integrating Herbs into Daily Life

Incorporating herbal medicine into daily life doesn't have to be complex. It can be as simple as drinking herbal teas, using herbal supplements, or cooking with fresh herbs. The key is consistency and mindfulness, paying attention to how your body responds and adjusting accordingly.

- **Herbal Teas:** A simple and enjoyable way to incorporate herbs. Teas made from red raspberry leaf, chamomile, or nettle offer gentle support for women's health.
- **Culinary Herbs:** Many common kitchen herbs, such as garlic, ginger, and turmeric, have potent health benefits. Incorporating them into meals can boost nutrition and support overall well-being.
- **Topical Applications:** Herbs can also be used externally in baths, oils, or salves to soothe skin conditions, relieve pain, or promote relaxation.

The Role of Herbs in Women's Health

Women's bodies go through unique cycles and changes, from menstruation to menopause. Herbal medicine offers a way to support these transitions naturally, providing relief from symptoms and supporting the body's inherent healing processes. Whether it's managing menstrual cramps with cramp bark, supporting fertility with Vitex, or easing menopause symptoms with black cohosh, herbs offer a versatile and gentle option for care.

The foundation of herbal medicine for women is built on understanding the intricate relationship between our bodies and the natural world. It's about recognizing the power of plants to heal and support and learning how to use this power wisely and respectfully.

CHAPTER 2: HERBS FOR MENSTRUAL HEALTH

The menstrual cycle, a natural part of a woman's life, can often bring discomfort and disruption. Yet, a compassionate and practical approach to easing these challenges lies within herbal medicine. This chapter explores the gentle power of herbs in supporting menstrual health, offering natural solutions for common issues such as menstrual cramps, premenstrual syndrome (PMS), and irregular cycles.

Easing Menstrual Cramps with Herbal Remedies

Menstrual cramps, or dysmenorrhea, can range from mild discomfort to severe pain, affecting daily activities and overall quality of life. Herbal remedies offer a soothing alternative to over-the-counter pain medications, targeting the root causes of discomfort with fewer side effects.

- **Cramp Bark (Viburnum opulus):** Aptly named, cramp bark is renowned for its antispasmodic properties, helping to relax muscle tension and ease cramping. A tea or tincture taken a few days before menstruation can be particularly beneficial.
- **Ginger (Zingiber officinale):** Ginger is a warming herb that not only soothes cramps but also addresses nausea sometimes associated with menstruation. Its anti-inflammatory properties make it a versatile remedy, easily incorporated into the diet as a tea, meal, or supplement.

- **Chamomile (Matricaria recutita):** Known for its calming effects, chamomile can relieve menstrual cramps and soothe the nervous system, promoting relaxation during discomfort.

Natural Solutions for PMS: Mood, Bloating, and Fatigue

Premenstrual syndrome encompasses a wide range of symptoms, including mood swings, bloating, and fatigue, affecting many women in the days leading up to menstruation.

- **Evening Primrose Oil (Oenothera biennis):** Rich in gamma-linolenic acid (GLA), evening primrose oil can help balance hormones and reduce PMS symptoms, particularly mood swings and breast tenderness.
- **Dandelion (Taraxacum officinale):** Dandelion acts as a natural diuretic, helping to relieve the bloating and water retention often associated with PMS. Its leaves can be consumed in salads or as a tea.
- **St. John's Wort (Hypericum perforatum):** Particularly effective for mood-related PMS symptoms, St. John's Wort should be used cautiously, as it can interact with other medications.

Regulating Menstrual Cycles Holistically

Irregular menstrual cycles can be a source of frustration and concern. While underlying health issues should always be addressed with a healthcare provider, certain herbs can support regularity and hormonal balance.

- **Vitex (Vitex agnus-castus):** Also known as chasteberry, Vitex is one of the most widely used herbs for menstrual cycle regulation. It works by balancing hormone levels, particularly progesterone, helping to regularize the menstrual cycle.
- **Maca (Lepidium meyenii):** Grown in the high Andes, Maca is a root vegetable that enhances energy, stamina, and hormone balance, supporting overall menstrual health.

- **Red Raspberry Leaf (Rubus idaeus):** Often associated with pregnancy, red raspberry leaf is also beneficial for menstrual health, helping to tone the uterine muscles and regulate cycles.

The journey through menstrual health challenges can be significantly eased with the thoughtful incorporation of herbal remedies. By tuning into the body's natural rhythms and supporting these healing herbs, women can navigate their menstrual cycles with greater comfort and balance. Remember, the key is to listen to your body, observe how it responds to different herbs, and adjust your approach as needed. This chapter is not just about treating symptoms but about embracing a holistic view of health, where the natural wisdom of the body and the healing power of plants work in harmony.

CHAPTER 3: EMBRACING PREGNANCY AND POSTPARTUM WITH HERBS

Pregnancy and the postpartum period are times of profound change and adaptation for women, both physically and emotionally. Herbs offer supportive care during these transformative months with their gentle strength and natural healing properties. This chapter delves into how to safely use herbs to alleviate pregnancy discomforts, prepare for labor and delivery, and support recovery and lactation in the postpartum period.

Safe Herbs for Nausea Relief and Nutritional Support

Morning sickness and nutritional needs significantly mark the pregnancy journey. Herbs can offer a soothing touch for nausea while providing vital nutrients for both mother and baby.

- **Ginger (Zingiber officinale):** A renowned remedy for nausea, ginger can be taken as a tea, in capsules, or even chewed as candied ginger. Its warming and soothing properties can help ease morning sickness.
- **Peppermint (Mentha piperita):** Peppermint tea is a gentle way to relieve nausea and digestive discomfort during pregnancy. Its refreshing flavor also makes it a pleasing option.
- **Red Raspberry Leaf (Rubus idaeus):** Rich in vitamins and minerals, red raspberry leaf is particularly beneficial in the second and third trimesters. It's known to strengthen uterine muscles, aiding labor preparation,

though it's best to consult a healthcare provider before starting.

Herbal Preparations for Labor and Delivery

As the due date approaches, certain herbs can help prepare the body for labor, promoting a smoother delivery.

- **Dates (Phoenix dactylifera):** While not an herb, dates have been studied for their positive effects on labor. Consuming dates in the weeks leading up to labor can promote cervical dilation and reduce the need for induced labor.
- **Evening Primrose Oil (Oenothera biennis):** Topically or orally, evening primrose oil can help soften the cervix and prepare the body for labor. It's typically recommended in the final weeks of pregnancy.

Nurturing Recovery: Postpartum Herbs for Healing and Lactation

The postpartum period, or the fourth trimester, is a time for healing and adjustment. Herbs can support physical recovery, emotional well-being, and lactation.

- **Nettle (Urtica dioica):** Rich in iron and vitamins, nettle is an excellent tonic for postpartum recovery. It supports energy levels and helps replenish nutrients lost during childbirth.
- **Fenugreek (Trigonella foenum-graecum):** Widely recognized for its lactation support, fenugreek can help increase milk supply. However, it should be used under the guidance of a healthcare provider, as it's not suitable for everyone.
- **Calendula (Calendula officinalis):** External calendula can help heal perineal tears or C-section scars. Its gentle, soothing properties support skin healing.

Embracing pregnancy and postpartum with herbs provides a natural pathway to support the body's journey through these life-changing experiences. While herbs offer gentle and practical support, it's crucial to approach herbal use during pregnancy and postpartum with care, always consulting with healthcare providers to ensure safety for both mother and baby.

CHAPTER 4: NAVIGATING MENOPAUSE WITH HERBAL ALLIES

Menopause, a natural transition in a woman's life, marks the end of her menstrual cycle. It's a period characterized by significant hormonal changes that can impact physical health, emotional well-being, and overall quality of life. Fortunately, nature offers a bounty of herbal allies that can help women navigate this transition more comfortably. This chapter explores how herbs can be used to mitigate common menopausal symptoms, support emotional health, and maintain hormonal balance and bone health.

Cooling Herbs for Hot Flashes and Night Sweats

Hot flashes and night sweats are among the most common and uncomfortable symptoms of menopause. Several herbs have been traditionally used to provide a cooling effect and reduce the frequency and intensity of these episodes.

- **Black Cohosh (Actaea racemosa):** Black cohosh has a long history of use for relieving menopausal symptoms and scorching flashes. It's thought to work by influencing serotonin receptors and improving vasomotor symptoms.
- **Sage (Salvia officinalis):** Sage tea has been traditionally consumed to reduce sweating and is specifically helpful for night sweats. Its estrogenic compounds may help balance hormones naturally.
- **Red Clover (Trifolium pratense):** Rich in isoflavones, red clover has

been studied for its potential to ease hot flashes. It's believed to act as a phytoestrogen, gently supporting hormonal balance during menopause.

Herbal Support for Emotional Well-being and Sleep

The emotional rollercoaster and sleep disturbances that often accompany menopause can significantly impact daily life. Certain herbs offer calming and soothing properties that can help improve mood and promote restful sleep.

- **St. John's Wort (Hypericum perforatum):** Known for its antidepressant properties, St. John's Wort can be beneficial for the mood swings and depression that some women experience during menopause. Caution is advised due to its interactions with various medications.
- **Valerian (Valeriana officinalis):** Valerian root is a well-known herbal sedative that helps to improve sleep quality and ease insomnia associated with menopause.
- **Passionflower (Passiflora incarnata):** Passionflower can alleviate anxiety and insomnia, promoting a sense of calm and making it easier to fall and stay asleep.

Maintaining Hormonal Balance and Bone Health

Hormonal fluctuations during menopause can affect bone density, increasing the risk of osteoporosis. Certain herbs and lifestyle and dietary changes can support hormonal balance and bone health.

- **Dong Quai (Angelica sinensis):** Often referred to as "female ginseng," Dong Quai is used in Traditional Chinese Medicine to support overall hormonal balance. It's believed to have phytoestrogenic effects, although research is mixed.
- **Horsetail (Equisetum arvense):** Rich in silica, horsetail can support bone density and health. It's often recommended as a part of a holistic approach to preventing or treating osteoporosis.

- **Vitex (Vitex agnus-castus):** While more commonly associated with menstrual health, Vitex can also support hormonal balance through menopause, particularly in the early stages.

Menopause is a significant phase in a woman's life, marking the transition into a period of wisdom and maturity. While it can come with challenges, the herbal world offers a treasure trove of allies to ease the journey. By tapping into the power of these plants, women can find natural relief from menopausal symptoms, support their emotional well-being, and maintain their health and vitality. As with any herbal regimen, it's essential to consult with a healthcare provider, especially during such a transformative time as menopause, to ensure the choices you make are safe and tailored to your unique health needs.

CHAPTER 5: HERBS FOR WOMEN'S OVERALL WELL-BEING

In the holistic wellness journey, herbs play a pivotal role, especially for women seeking to nurture their health across various spectrums of life. This chapter dives into the heart of herbal wisdom, exploring how certain herbs can bolster energy, reduce stress, enhance immunity, address chronic conditions, and seamlessly integrate into daily routines for optimal health.

Herbs for Energy, Stress Reduction, and Immunity

In today's fast-paced world, maintaining energy levels, managing stress, and keeping the immune system strong is crucial for overall well-being. Nature offers an array of herbs that meet these needs with grace and potency.

- **Ashwagandha (Withania somnifera):** Known as an adaptogen, ashwagandha helps the body adapt to stress and conserves energy. Modulating the stress response supports sustained energy throughout the day without the jitters associated with stimulants.
- **Rhodiola (Rhodiola rosea):** Another adaptogenic hero enhances physical and mental energy and endurance. It's particularly beneficial during stress or fatigue, helping to uplift mood and combat burnout.
- **Echinacea (Echinacea spp.):** Widely recognized for its immune-boosting properties, Echinacea can help prevent and ease the duration of colds, making it a staple in the natural wellness toolkit.

Herbal Strategies for Chronic Conditions Affecting Women

Certain chronic conditions disproportionately affect women, such as autoimmune diseases, thyroid disorders, and osteoporosis. Herbs, alongside conventional treatments, can offer supportive care.

- **Turmeric (Curcuma longa):** The active compound in turmeric, curcumin, has potent anti-inflammatory and antioxidant properties, making it beneficial for conditions like rheumatoid arthritis and other inflammatory disorders.
- **Bladderwrack (Fucus vesiculosus):** Rich in iodine, bladderwrack supports thyroid health, particularly for those with hypothyroidism. However, it should be used under the guidance of a healthcare professional to ensure proper dosage and avoid iodine excess.
- **Nettle (Urtica dioica):** Nettle's high mineral content, particularly calcium and magnesium, supports bone health, making it a valuable herb for preventing and managing osteoporosis.

Integrating Herbs into Daily Life for Optimal Health

Incorporating herbs into one's daily routine doesn't require drastic changes but relatively small, intentional additions that enhance wellness.

- **Cooking with Culinary Herbs:** Incorporate rosemary, thyme, and garlic into your meals. Not only do they elevate the flavor of dishes, but they also contribute antioxidants and health-promoting compounds.
- **Herbal Teas as Daily Rituals:** Create a daily ritual around herbal teas. A morning cup of green tea offers a gentle caffeine boost along with antioxidants, while a nightly chamomile tea can soothe the mind and prepare the body for rest.
- **Topical Herbal Applications:** Explore using herbal-infused oils or lotions for skin health or muscle relaxation. Lavender oil, for example, can be

massaged into temples to alleviate stress or added to bathwater for a calming soak.

Herbs offer a profound yet gentle means to support and enhance women's well-being across all facets of life. From boosting energy and managing stress to fortifying immunity and addressing chronic conditions, the plant kingdom provides a wealth of resources for those willing to explore and integrate its bounty into their daily routines. Embracing herbal wisdom nurtures the body and fosters a deeper connection with nature, leading to a balanced and vibrant life. Remember, the journey towards optimal health is personal and holistic, with herbs serving as companions and guides.

CHAPTER 6: BEAUTY AND SKINCARE: THE HERBAL WAY

In beauty and skincare, the allure of herbal remedies lies not just in their natural essence but in their profound ability to nourish, heal, and rejuvenate from within. This chapter unfolds the secrets of using herbs to enhance beauty, presenting a holistic approach to skincare and hair care that aligns with nature's rhythms and our ancestors' wisdom.

Herbs for Glowing Skin: Cleansers, Toners, and Moisturizers

The foundation of radiant skin lies in a balanced regimen of cleansing, toning, and moisturizing—a ritual that can be beautifully enriched with herbal infusions.

- **Cleansers:** Aloe vera, known for its soothing and hydrating properties, is an excellent base in herbal cleansers. Combine it with antimicrobial herbs like neem or tea tree oil for acne-prone skin or chamomile and calendula for sensitive skin to gently cleanse without stripping the skin's natural oils.
- **Toners:** Witch hazel, infused with lavender or rose petals, acts as a gentle toner that balances the skin's pH, tightens pores, and prepares the skin for moisturizing. Its anti-inflammatory properties soothe irritation and redness, leaving the skin refreshed.

- **Moisturizers:** For a deeply nourishing moisturizer, blend shea butter with herbal oils such as rosehip for its regenerative properties, frankincense for its ability to reduce the appearance of scars and wrinkles, and geranium for its balancing effect on sebum production. This concoction hydrates, heals, and rejuvenates the skin at a cellular level.

Natural Hair Care: Strength and Shine from Roots to Ends

Herbal remedies can transform hair care into a nurturing ritual that strengthens and revitalizes the hair from roots to ends.

- **Scalp Treatments:** Rosemary and peppermint essential oils stimulate the scalp, promoting blood circulation and hair growth. Infuse these into a carrier oil like coconut or jojoba for a rejuvenating scalp massage that energizes hair follicles for more robust growth.
- **Herbal Rinses:** Chamomile tea brightens blonde hair, while a sage or black tea rinse can deepen darker hues. Nettle and horsetail (rich in silica) strengthen the hair, reducing breakage and promoting shine.
- **Deep Conditioning Treatments:** Avocado and olive oils, enriched with ylang-ylang or lavender essential oils, create luxurious deep conditioning treatments that restore moisture and elasticity, leaving hair soft, shiny, and healthy.

Anti-Aging Herbs: Nourishing Skin from Within

Aging gracefully is about nurturing the skin from within and embracing herbs known for their antioxidant, regenerative, and protective qualities.

- **Antioxidant Powerhouses:** Green tea and turmeric are rich in antioxidants that protect the skin from free radical damage, one of the primary causes of premature aging. Incorporating these herbs into your diet or skincare routine can help maintain the skin's elasticity and youthful glow.
- **Collagen Boosters:** Gotu kola and sea buckthorn are revered for their

ability to boost collagen production, enhancing the skin's firmness and reducing the appearance of fine lines and wrinkles.

· **Skin Protectors:** Ginkgo biloba and milk thistle protect the skin against environmental stressors and pollution thanks to their potent antioxidant profiles. Their inclusion in skincare formulations or as dietary supplements can shield the skin from the elements, preserving its health and vitality.

Embracing the herbal way in beauty and skincare isn't just about tapping into nature's bounty—it's a commitment to nurturing ourselves with the gentleness and wisdom inherent in the earth's offerings. By integrating herbs into our skincare and haircare routines, we not only bestow upon ourselves the gift of natural beauty but also forge a deeper connection with the environment, celebrating the timeless bond between nature and nurture. As we explore these herbal remedies, let us remember that true beauty flourishes from within—a radiant reflection of health, happiness, and harmony with the natural world.

CHAPTER 7: CRAFTING YOUR HERBAL TOOLKIT

Embarking on a health and wellness journey through herbal medicine isn't just about understanding the properties and benefits of various herbs. It's also about acquiring the skills and knowledge to craft your remedies and even grow the herbs that will become part of your wellness regimen. This chapter is dedicated to empowering you with the practical know-how to make herbal teas, tinctures, topicals, and tips for cultivating your own women's health herb garden.

Making Herbal Teas, Tinctures, and Topicals

Herbal Teas: Making teas is the most straightforward way to start using herbs. Herbal teas are therapeutic and provide a moment of peace in your day. To make a tea, steep 1-2 teaspoons of dried herb (or 2-3 teaspoons of fresh herb) in a cup of boiling water for 5-10 minutes. Prepare an infusion for a more substantial medicinal effect by steeping a more significant amount of herb in a covered vessel for several hours or overnight. Chamomile for relaxation, peppermint for digestion, and nettle for its nutrient-rich profile are great starters.

Tinctures are concentrated herbal extracts from soaking herbs in alcohol or vinegar. They are potent and long-lasting, making them valuable to your herbal toolkit. To make a tincture:

1. Fill a jar one-third to one-half full with dried herbs, then pour enough alcohol (vodka or brandy works well) to cover the herbs completely.
2. Seal the jar and let it sit in a cool, dark place for 4-6 weeks, shaking it every few days.
3. Strain the mixture through cheesecloth, and store the liquid in amber dropper bottles for easy use.

Topicals: Herbal topicals, including salves and balms, are excellent for treating skin issues, aches, and pains. To make a simple salve, infuse oils (such as olive or coconut oil) with herbs like calendula for skin healing or arnica for bruises and sore muscles. Gently heat the infused oil with beeswax until the wax melts, then pour the mixture into containers to cool. As it solidifies, you'll have a nourishing herbal salve.

Growing Your Own Women's Health Herb Garden

Cultivating an herb garden tailored to women's health provides you with fresh, potent herbs at your fingertips and deepens your connection to the healing power of nature. Many medicinal herbs are easy to grow, whether you have a spacious backyard or a small balcony.

1. **Selecting Herbs:** Choose herbs that resonate with your specific health needs and thrive in your climate. Consider starting with versatile herbs like lavender (for relaxation and skin health), lemon balm (for stress and sleep), and yarrow (for menstrual health and wound healing).
2. **Planting:** Most herbs prefer well-draining soil and plenty of sunshine. While many herbs are forgiving and can grow in less-than-ideal conditions, giving them a good start will ensure they thrive. Research each herb's specific needs regarding soil, water, and sunlight.
3. **Care and Harvesting:** Regularly tending to your herbs by watering them as needed and harvesting them correctly will keep them healthy and productive. Harvest herbs in the morning when their essential oil content is highest. Always leave enough of the plant so it can continue to grow.

4. **Sustainability:** Consider companion planting to attract beneficial insects and repel pests naturally. Composting and using natural fertilizers will keep your garden and herbs healthy and sustainable.

Creating your herbal toolkit and growing your herb garden are enriching practices that enhance your self-sufficiency and deepen your engagement with the natural world. As you learn to craft teas, tinctures, and topicals from the herbs you've nurtured with your own hands, you'll develop a more intuitive understanding of their properties and potential. This hands-on approach brings the power of herbal medicine into your daily life and fosters a profound connection with the earth, empowering you to take charge of your health and well-being in the most natural way possible.

CHAPTER 8: RECIPES AND REMEDIES

Embarking on a self-care journey through herbalism is a deeply personal and enriching experience. It's about more than just addressing health issues—it's about nurturing your body and soul with the gifts of the earth. This chapter brings you closer to this goal, offering a collection of herbal recipes and remedies specifically designed for women's health issues, alongside DIY beauty and skincare recipes to enhance your natural glow.

Herbal Recipes for Women's Health Issues

Cramp Relief Tea Blend

- Ingredients: 1 part cramp bark, 1 part chamomile flowers, 1 part ginger root.
- Instructions: Combine the herbs in a tea infuser. Pour boiling water over the herbs and steep for 15 minutes. Drink up to three times a day during menstruation to ease cramps and soothe discomfort.

Mood-Balancing Tincture

- Ingredients: 1 part St. John's Wort, 1 part Vitex berries, vodka.
- Instructions: Fill a jar one-third with the dried herbs and then cover completely with vodka. Seal and store in a cool, dark place for 4-6 weeks, shaking daily. Strain and take 1-2 droppers complete daily, or as needed, to help balance mood swings associated with PMS or menopause.

Fertility Support Infusion

- Ingredients: 1 part red raspberry leaf, 1 part nettle leaf, 1/2 part peppermint leaf.
- Instructions: Mix herbs. Use one heaping tablespoon per cup of boiling water and steep for 20 minutes. Drink 1-2 cups daily to support fertility and uterine health.

DIY Herbal Beauty and Skincare Recipes

Herbal Facial Steam for Glowing Skin

- Ingredients: 1 part lavender, 1 part rose petals, 1 part chamomile.
- Instructions: Combine herbs in a large bowl. Pour boiling water over the herbs and lean over the bowl with a towel over your head to trap the steam. Enjoy the steam for 5-10 minutes for a soothing, detoxifying facial that leaves your skin radiant.

Nourishing Hair Rinse for Shine and Strength

- Ingredients: 1 part rosemary, 1 part sage, apple cider vinegar.
- Instructions: Steep the herbs in boiling water for 30 minutes. Strain and add to an equal part of apple cider vinegar. Use as a final rinse after shampooing to stimulate hair growth, enhance shine, and strengthen the hair.

Anti-Aging Skin Serum

- Ingredients: 1 part rosehip seed oil, 1 part evening primrose oil, vitamin E oil, essential oils of lavender and frankincense.
- Instructions: Mix the oils, adding a few drops of vitamin E and essential oils for every ounce of base oil. Apply nightly to clean, damp skin. The blend contains antioxidants and essential fatty acids, promoting skin

regeneration and elasticity.

Herbal Support for Hormonal Balance

Vitex Elixir:

- **Ingredients:** 1 part Vitex berries, 5 parts alcohol (vodka or brandy), 5 parts water.
- **Instructions:** Combine Vitex berries with alcohol and water in a jar. Seal tightly and store in a cool, dark place for 4 weeks, shaking daily. Strain the mixture, and take 1-2 droppers each morning to help regulate hormonal imbalances and support menstrual health.

Natural Remedies for Anxiety and Stress

Lemon Balm and Lavender Tea:

- **Ingredients:** 1 teaspoon dried lemon balm, 1 teaspoon dried lavender flowers, 1 cup boiling water.
- **Instructions:** Place the herbs in a teapot or cup. Pour boiling water over them and steep for 10 minutes. Strain and enjoy this calming tea during moments of stress or before bedtime to promote relaxation and peaceful sleep.

Support for Digestive Health

Peppermint and Ginger Digestive Aid:

- **Ingredients:** ½ teaspoon dried peppermint leaves, ½ teaspoon grated fresh ginger, 1 cup boiling water.
- **Instructions:** Combine peppermint and ginger in a mug. Pour boiling water over the herbs and let steep for 10 minutes. Drink after meals to aid digestion, soothe the stomach, and relieve bloating.

Enhancing Fertility

Red Raspberry Leaf and Nettle Fertility Tea:

- **Ingredients:** 1 part red raspberry leaf, 1 part nettle leaf, ½ part peppermint leaf, boiling water.
- **Instructions:** Blend the herbs. Use one tablespoon of the herbal mix per cup of boiling water. Steep for 15 minutes, strain, and drink 1-2 cups daily. This tea is rich in vitamins and minerals, supporting overall reproductive health and enhancing fertility.

Menopause Symptom Relief

Sage and Black Cohosh Cooling Spray:

- **Ingredients:** 1 teaspoon dried sage, 1 teaspoon dried black cohosh, 1 cup distilled water, spray bottle.
- **Instructions:** Boil water and pour over the herbs. Allow to steep until cool, then strain into a spray bottle. Use as a cooling mist to relieve hot flashes and night sweats. Store in the refrigerator for an extra cooling effect.

Breast Health Massage Oil

Dandelion and Flaxseed Massage Oil:

- **Ingredients:** ¼ cup dandelion infused oil, ¼ cup flaxseed oil, 10 drops of frankincense essential oil, dark glass bottle.
- **Instructions:** Mix the oils and store them in a dark glass bottle. Use the oil to gently massage the breast area in a circular motion, moving towards the armpits to promote lymphatic drainage and support breast health.

These recipes and remedies are just the beginning of what's possible when you harness the power of herbs for health and beauty. Each one invites you to engage with the natural world, experimenting and learning what works best for your unique body and needs. Whether you're seeking relief from health issues or looking to enhance your natural beauty, remember that the most potent medicine and the most effective beauty treatments are often those that come from the earth, prepared by your own hands with intention and care. As you integrate these herbal practices into your life, you'll find healing and rejuvenation, a deeper connection to the rhythms of nature, and a greater sense of harmony within yourself.

CONCLUSION

Embracing Herbal Harmony for Life-Long Women's Health

As we draw the curtains on this enlightening journey through the world of herbal medicine tailored for women, we must reflect on the profound connection we've rekindled with nature and our bodies. Embracing herbal harmony isn't merely about using plants to address health concerns; it's about nurturing a lifelong relationship with the natural world and recognizing the deep wisdom it offers for our health, well-being, and overall vitality.

The Path to Wholeness

Herbal medicine serves as a bridge to our ancestral past, a time when humans lived in close harmony with the earth, intuitively understanding the healing powers of plants. By incorporating herbs into our daily lives, we tap into this ancient wisdom and take an active role in our health and wellness. This journey is about more than finding natural alternatives; it's about embracing a holistic approach to living that honors the interconnectedness of mind, body, and spirit.

A Personalized Journey

Every woman's path to health and well-being is unique and shaped by her experiences, challenges, and needs. Herbal medicine respects this individuality, offering many options that can be tailored to each person. Whether navigating menstrual health, embracing the changes of menopause, or seeking natural beauty remedies, the herbal world is rich with possibilities. The key is listening to your body, nature, and the subtle shifts that occur as you incorporate herbs into your life.

Empowerment Through Knowledge

Knowledge is power, especially when taking charge of your health. By learning about herbs and how to use them safely and effectively, you empower yourself to make informed decisions about your well-being. This book has aimed to equip you with the knowledge you need to begin this journey, but the learning continues beyond here. Continue to explore, experiment, and educate yourself. Remember, herbal harmony is a lifelong journey of discovery and growth.

The Healing Power of Nature

At the heart of herbal medicine is a deep respect for the healing power of nature. It's a reminder that, amidst the hustle and bustle of modern life, we are part of something much larger and more beautiful. By aligning ourselves with the rhythms of nature, we find a sense of balance and peace that transcends physical health. This connection to the natural world is healing, offering a sanctuary for the soul and the body.

Moving Forward with Grace

As we move forward, let us carry with us the lessons and insights gained from the pages of this book. Let herbal harmony guide us, not just in times of illness, but as a foundation for living a life of vitality, beauty, and wellness. Embrace the plants and their wisdom, let them nurture and sustain you, and walk the path of health and wholeness with grace and gratitude.

In conclusion, embracing herbal harmony for life-long women's health is a journey back to our roots, to a way of living that is in tune with the natural world. It's a call to embrace the gentle yet profound power of plants, weave their magic into our daily lives, and celebrate the female body's incredible resilience and strength. May your journey be filled with health, harmony, and the healing embrace of nature.

APPENDICES

The journey into herbal medicine is rewarding and complex, requiring an understanding of safety, a commitment to continued education, and familiarity with the herbs. These appendices serve as a guide to navigating these waters with confidence and curiosity.

Herb Safety and Dosage Guidelines

Herbal medicine offers natural healing options but must be approached with respect and knowledge. Understanding herbs' safety and proper dosages is paramount to ensuring their benefits can be enjoyed without adverse effects.

- **Consultation:** Always consult with a healthcare professional before starting any new herbal regimen, especially if you are pregnant, nursing, or taking prescription medications.
- **Dosage:** Start with the lowest recommended dose and observe your body's response. Dosages vary widely based on the herb, its form (tincture, tea, capsule), and the individual.
- **Quality:** Use high-quality, organic herbs from reputable sources to ensure purity and potency.
- **Allergies:** Be aware of potential allergic reactions. If you're trying a new herb, start with a small amount to monitor your body's response.
- **Side Effects:** Educate yourself on the possible side effects of herbs. Discontinue use and consult a healthcare provider if adverse reactions occur.

Glossary of Common Herbs and Their Uses

Ashwagandha (Withania somnifera): An adaptogen known for its ability to reduce stress and anxiety, improve energy levels, and support overall wellness.

Chamomile (Matricaria recutita): A gentle herb famous for its calming effects, aiding sleep, and soothing digestive issues.

Echinacea (Echinacea spp.): Used to boost the immune system and fight off colds and flu.

Ginger (Zingiber officinale): A warming herb that aids digestion, relieves nausea and has anti-inflammatory properties.

Lavender (Lavandula angustifolia): Known for its relaxing aroma, lavender is used to reduce anxiety, improve sleep, and heal skin irritations.

Nettle (Urtica dioica): Rich in nutrients, nettle supports joint health, urinary function, and allergy relief.

Peppermint (Mentha piperita): Offers relief from digestive discomfort and headaches and has energizing properties.

Turmeric (Curcuma longa): Contains curcumin, a compound with potent anti-inflammatory and antioxidant effects.

Valerian (Valeriana officinalis): A root used for its soothing properties, helping with insomnia and anxiety.

This glossary is a starting point. Each herb carries many benefits and potential applications, underscoring the richness of herbal medicine as a field of study and practice. As you continue to explore and learn, let these appendices serve as a foundation upon which you can build a deeper, more intuitive understanding of herbal wellness.

SOURCES

https://www.verywellhealth.com/herbs-for-menstrual-cramps-89901

https://www.jafariacupuncture.com/herbs-for-menstrual-cramps-top-10-best-herbs-for-relieving-cramps-during-menstruation/

https://www.naturopathy-uk.com/news/news-cnm-blog/blog/2022/03/28/6-must-use-herbs-to-balance-hormones/

https://www.gaiaherbs.com/blogs/seeds-of-knowledge/natural-solutions-menstrual-cramps

https://naturveda.fr/en/blogs/actus-sante/relieve-menstrual-pain-plant-grace

https://woashwellness.com/a/blog/herbs-for-pregnancy

https://hearttherapeutics.com.au/blogs/news/herbs-and-herbal-teas-for-pregnancy-and-beyond

https://americanpregnancy.org/healthy-pregnancy/is-it-safe/herbal-tea/

https://wingedwellness.com/blogs/mind-body/7-herbs-for-menopause

https://www.healthline.com/nutrition/menopause-herbs#3.-Dong-quai

https://www.everydayhealth.com/menopause/promising-supplements-for-menopausal-symptoms/

https://menoveda.com/blogs/knowledge/ayurvedic-herbs-that-are-a-boon-for-menopause

https://www.quinessence.com/blog/herbal-way-smoother-skin

https://www.healthline.com/health/beauty-skin-care/natural-skin-care-routine

https://blog.mountainroseherbs.com/building-a-herbal-starter-kit

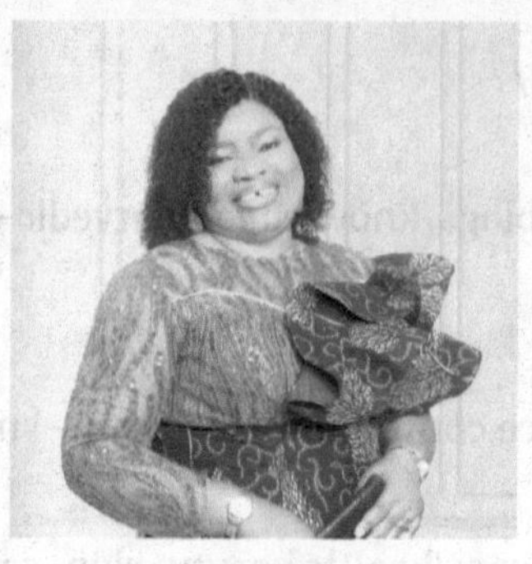

About the Author

Glorioustina Essia is a multifaceted professional whose expertise traverses the realms of technology, artificial intelligence, literature, and natural health. As a driving force in artificial intelligence, particularly in prompt engineering, she has established herself as a pioneer. Her proficiency extends to project management, network marketing, website development, and copywriting, showcasing a unique blend of technical understanding and creative flair.

A prolific author and publisher, Glorioustina's literary works span multiple genres, captivating a diverse audience with her narrative skill and inspiring a new generation of writers to unlock their creative potential. Her passion for storytelling matches her commitment to exploring and advocating for holistic health practices. Renowned in herbal medicine, she dedicates her life to studying and promoting natural health.

Glorioustina Essia's professional and personal journey is characterized by an unwavering dedication to her core strengths and a ceaseless pursuit of knowledge. Her zeal and expertise embody the limitless possibilities that arise from a commitment to innovation, quality, and a deep-seated passion for understanding the future of technology and the ancient wisdom of herbal medicine. Glorioustina is a testament to the power of interdisciplinary knowledge and its impact in a world where technology, literature, and natural health converge.

Also by Glorioustina Essia

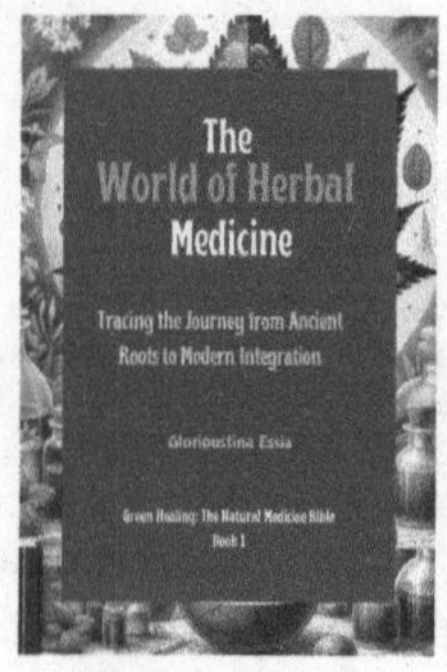

The World of Herbal Medicine

In an era where the rush of modern medicine often overshadows the pursuit of holistic health, the timeless wisdom of herbal remedies remains largely untapped. Do you find yourself seeking a more natural approach to health and wellness yet still determining where to begin or how to integrate these practices with modern healthcare?

Embark on a transformative journey with Book 1 of "Green Healing: The Natural Medicine Bible": "The World of Herbal Medicine." This enlightening volume takes you through the ancient pathways to the modern integration of herbal healing. Discover herbal medicine's rich history and evolution across different cultures, including the profound insights of Traditional Chinese Medicine, Ayurveda, and indigenous practices. Unravel how herbalism has evolved through historical epochs and how it beautifully intersects with modern medical practices today.

Embrace the journey to holistic health – add this captivating volume to your collection and begin exploring the world of herbal medicine today!

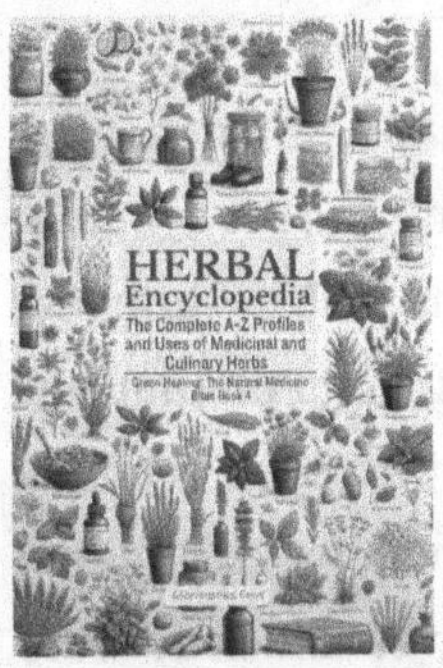

Herbal Encyclopedia

Embark on a journey through nature's apothecary with "Herbal Encyclopedia: The Complete A-Z Profiles and Uses of Medicinal and Culinary Herbs." This guide unravels the secrets of herbs, from age-old medicinal uses to enhancing culinary delights. Each page introduces you to a new herb, revealing its history, health benefits, and how it can be incorporated into your daily life. Whether you're a budding herbalist or a seasoned enthusiast, this encyclopedia offers easy-to-understand profiles, practical tips, and a connection to the ancient art of herbal healing.

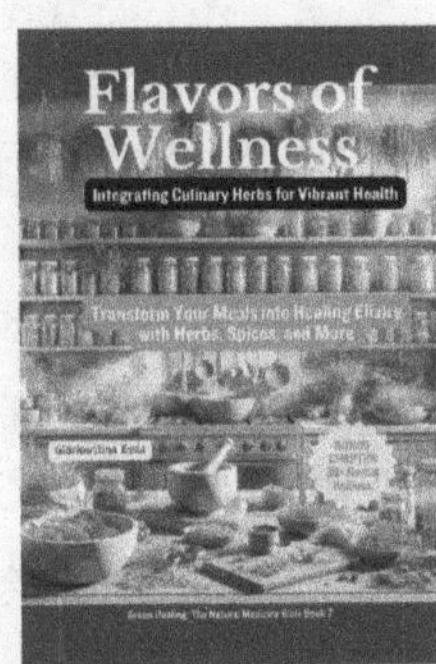

Flavors of Wellness

This guide invites you into a world where every herb in your garden or kitchen pantry is a key to unlocking vibrant health and elevating your culinary creations. From basil-infused breakfasts to rosemary-laced dinners, discover how to weave the magic of herbs into everyday cooking. Learn to grow, harvest, and preserve your herbs, ensuring your dishes burst with flavor and nutritional benefits all year round. Whether you're a novice cook or a seasoned chef, this book offers simple, delicious ways to incorporate healing herbs into your daily diet. Embrace the herbal lifestyle—where wellness and flavor live harmoniously on your plate.

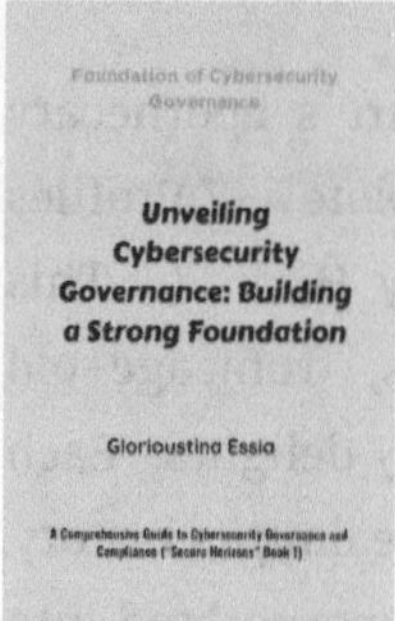

Unveiling Cybersecurity Governance

In the ever-expanding digital landscape, safeguarding sensitive information and maintaining robust cybersecurity practices have become paramount. "Unveiling Cybersecurity Governance: Building a Strong Foundation" is a comprehensive guide that delves into cybersecurity governance's core principles and components, equipping readers with the knowledge and tools to establish a secure digital environment.

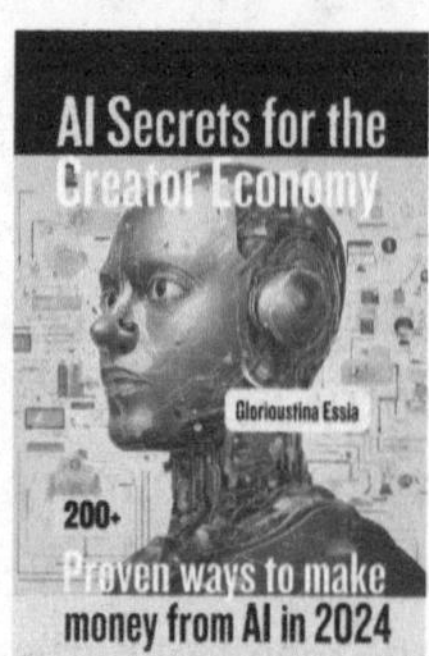

AI Secrets for the Creator Economy: 200+ Proven ways to make money from AI in 2024

In a world driven by innovation and transformation, the Creator Economy emerges as a powerful force, with Artificial Intelligence (AI) at its beating heart. This book, "AI Secrets for the Creator Economy: 200+ Proven Ways to Make Money from AI in 2024 and Beyond," is more than just a book; it's your key to unlocking the incredible synergy between AI and creativity, opening the door to a wealth of opportunities for those who are willing to seize them.